THE INNER WARRIOR

THE POWER WITHIN

WAYNE FORREST

The Inner Warrior
Published by Wayne Forrest 2024 Copyright © 2024

ISBN 978-0-473-71599-1 paperback

Publishing and printing services supplied by
PublishMe, New Plymouth, New Zealand
www.publishme.co.nz

ENDORSEMENT

"In a world filled with uncertainty and doubt, *'The Inner Warrior: The Power Within'* serves as a beacon of hope and inspiration. Wayne offers a compelling roadmap for self- discovery and personal growth, reminding us that our greatest strength lies within. This book is a powerful reminder that with determination and belief in oneself, anything is possible."

— Mary Morrissey, bestselling author of *The Field of Dreams & Brave Thinking: The Art and Science of Creating a Life You Love*.

ACKNOWLEDGEMENTS

I want to express my deepest gratitude to all those who have
supported me along my journey.

Thank you to Jen Stoddart, an incredible person who has sadly passed from this human experience. Her profound knowledge of spinal injuries, her farming background, and her role as a personal caregiver and neighbor in the farming community of Mangaorapa, Porangahau, New Zealand, were invaluable. As an ex-physio, her accountability, coaching, and support during the early years of my spinal accident helped make my dream of farming post injury possible.

I am immensely grateful to my parents, Allen and Marilyn Forrest, for their unwavering support throughout my life. Their dedication to my upbringing instilled in me values of integrity, honesty, and a strong work ethic.

To Kathy, my wife, soul mate, muse, and best friend, thank you for walking with me on this wonderful journey and helping our dreams come true.

To my incredible children—Megan, Samantha, Jessica and Logan. Each of you has brought joy, wisdom, and purpose into my life, and I am profoundly grateful for the unique gifts you bring to our family. You bring immense joy to my heart and inspire me daily.

To my precious grandchildren: your laughter, curiosity, and boundless energy remind me of the beauty and wonder in the world. You have filled my heart with love.

INTRODUCTION

"In contrast to traditional masculine ego- driven order, the modern man stands rooted in self-truth, love, and curiosity. He wields physical strength not as a display but as an avenue to explore both body and mind."

In today's complex world, it's tough for a man to be himself amidst confusing narratives. While the emphasis on feminine energy is commendable, discussions often revolve around past missteps and prescriptions for how men should navigate today's world, where we can still be men and bring the masculine to this experience without the shame, anger, and embarrassment of perceived past wrongs. These wrongs are sometimes passed down from generations gone before us.

After dislocating my neck in a rugby game, a friend's visit inspired me to write this book. His words only the other week, praising my positivity after my life-changing accident, fuelled my belief in helping others with their mindset.

My positive mindset stems from my upbringing, during which my parents, always positive, focused on strengths rather than limitations.

Growing up on a farm in Hawke's Bay, New Zealand, instilled in me a sense of toughness and a can-do attitude. Farming was my first love. It was a community where people worked and played hard. They didn't show their feelings of sadness, weakness or anxiety — not in public, anyway.

This environment, while shaping my resilience,

also posed challenges, encouraging me to hide my feelings, especially during school bullying incidents that I felt I couldn't share with my parents. This pattern of hiding my feelings has repeated itself many times over the years.

At age twenty-five, I was at the peak of physical fitness when an accident during a rugby match dislocated my neck, robbing me of what I believed defined me. Once a man who ran everywhere, I now found myself unable to move limbs or perform basic tasks. To begin with, I couldn't feed myself or go to the bathroom without someone helping me.

Since that 1995 accident, my journey has been one of transformation whereby I discovered a profound inner strength fuelled by love for myself. This is a power we can all embrace in this ever-changing world. You will find that this new power still utilizes the physical strength you have as a man and retains your unique personality of what it is to be you, but along with that comes more fun and laughter, allowing you to harness it in a new way.

In contrast to traditional masculine ego-driven order, the modern man stands rooted in self-truth, love, and curiosity. He wields physical strength not as a display but as an avenue to explore both body and mind.

Ego is fighting hard to keep its grip on the world in which we live. A man with an over-developed ego tries his best to force everything in his outer world into order. The modern man, in contrast, will stand in a place of love in his own heart, not seeking the approval of others. He will stay curious and constantly question his own beliefs. He still physically lifts the heavy bags or digs the hole and builds the fence, but does it with fun and ease from a desire to experience his mind and body's full potential in all his achievements.

Perhaps like you, I felt powerless, confused and even angry, even before my accident, and at many different times during my life. For years I felt this way, with no idea why I felt so powerless. I knew there was something missing in my life.

I just didn't know what it was.

Until recently, there have been few alternatives for men to feel and learn to be powerful, but the following is my system for being powerful and having fun as you are doing it, too.

There's no competition to establish who's better or who's right. It's not about becoming soft or being more feminine. To truly empower ourselves, we must strike a balance between the masculine and feminine energies, steering clear of rigid stereotypes. It's about living into the full potential of both, fostering a new era of enlightened masculinity.

My wish for you is to uncover the transformative power within, enabling you to step confidently into today's world as an enlightened powerhouse. What the world truly needs is more men and women who have come alive!

CHAPTER 1

Belief!

"Believe NOTHING and question EVERYTHING."

"The seeds of every conflict, argument, and war are sown in belief systems."

Our lives are shaped by the beliefs we have. Whether rooted in Christianity, Islam, Judaism, atheism, or a belief in the higher self, the power of the Universe, or the wonders of science, these convictions define who we are. Additionally, societal beliefs — be they in the government, prevailing policies, or the shared values in our schools and by our family and friends
— contribute to the mosaic of our truths.

Consider this: everything we create in our world is born from belief, from the homes we build to the communities we form, from our schools to the cultures we embrace. A wise spiritual teacher once urged seekers to find their truth by embracing a mindset of curiosity and questioning, advising, "Believe NOTHING and question EVERYTHING."

Why? Because beliefs mold our powerful identity and can breed an 'us versus them' mentality. The seeds of every conflict, argument, and war are sown in belief systems. That's why, as you delve into the contents of this book, I encourage you to stay curious and challenge the ideas presented. What follows is my personal interpretation — an awareness of my extraordinary journey as a spiritual being having a human experience.

My truth, shared within these pages, is driven by a desire to inspire and transform. If this book resonates with just one person, nudging them to live their best life and contribute to making the world a better place, then my Inner Warrior compels me to share it. There's an unrelenting longing within me, a call from the soul that breathes life into me, urging me to share my insights. Strengthening my bond with my Inner Warrior amplifies this call, reinforcing the conviction to act and make a positive impact.

As I type these words, the excitement wells up within me — a sign that I am aligned with my true power, the Inner Warrior. Throughout this book, I will articulate my understanding of what the Inner Warrior means to me, then show you the process of connecting with it, and explore how this connection can create a life that is easier and infinitely more enjoyable.

CHAPTER 2

The Journey to Connection

"Breathe, Wayne, breathe!"

"You created this."

In my late twenties, anxiety started to creep into my life, manifesting in panic attacks that hit me hard, particularly when driving down the quiet country roads of the place I called home. One day, amid heart palpitations and loss of vision, I pulled over and gave myself a stern pep talk: "Breathe, Wayne, breathe!"

As I calmed down, a quiet, but calm voice from deep within whispered, "You are creating this." Confused, I asked, "What do you mean I am creating this?" The voice persisted without argument: "You created this."

It dawned on me that my thinking, specifically the *way* I was thinking, fuelled my anxiety. This revelation sparked a fascination with the power of thoughts and their ability to shape our reality — a journey that unfolded over the years.

Looking back, I now recognize that calm voice as my Inner Warrior. Some call it the higher self, spirit, or the God within, but I prefer Inner Warrior, as it resonates with me — confidence, courage, power, and strength.

Anxiety, much like anger, often stems from trauma. In my case, it traced back to the sporting accident when I was 25, dislocating my neck and injuring my spinal cord. I transformed from a tough farmer, scaling hills and handling cattle and sheep, to a man unable to move anything. The shift was drastic, and the reality of never walking again loomed over me.

I became a silent worrier, a product of my upbringing that discouraged the display of 'weakness'. Frustration and occasional anger replaced open communication as a young boy. It was then brought to the forefront of my consciousness with medical professionals telling me what could go wrong. Knowledge can be power, yet I obsessed over what may potentially happen, thus creating fear. Fear became a constant companion, evolving beyond health concerns to a pervasive anxiety that made even routine tasks daunting.

Driving again, two years post-accident, was a monumental milestone. It allowed me the freedom and independence to drive to social events and public places. Operating a machine called an Argo, adapted so I could drive it, I resumed the day- to-day management of the farm. Looking back, I marvel at the resilience required to face fear and anxiety daily, a battle unknown to those around me.

Silently grappling with my emotions, I concealed my struggles, adhering to the expectation of a tough New Zealand farmer. I told nobody, even those closest to me, as I felt shame for having fearful thoughts and feelings. If you're navigating similar challenges, battling fear and anxiety each day, give yourself credit. You're facing it head-on, so take a moment to celebrate by giving yourself a pat on the back. There's a better way, though, a light at the end of the tunnel, and you are on the right road.

I confess I was a Worrier, not a Warrior. Today, I predominantly live from my Inner Warrior, a source devoid of fear and anxiety, possessing foresight, wholeness, and a serene love for life.

Despite occasional slips into worry, I'm improving daily. My aspiration is to guide you towards a better way of living, transcending anxiety, fear, frustration, and anger to begin living a life for which you can truly feel grateful.

CHAPTER 3

Unveiling the Blueprint of Your Mind

"Its role is clear — to keep us safe. When it senses danger, our bodies respond with the familiar freeze, flight, or fight reaction."

Before we plunge deeper into unraveling the secrets of our Inner Warrior, let's shed light on the three fundamental aspects of our brain that played a pivotal role in my journey of understanding and overcoming anxiety and fear.

1. The Reptilian Brain — Our Sentinel of Safety

This ancient part of our brain has been on duty for millions of years, always on the lookout for danger. Stemming from our cave-dwelling ancestors, it prioritizes reproduction and survival. Back then, the saber-toothed tiger was our main threat, and swift reactions were essential for survival. Fast forward to today, where the threats have evolved but the Reptilian Brain hasn't much altered.

Its role is clear — to keep us safe. When it senses danger, our bodies respond with the familiar freeze, flight, or fight reaction. Some face it head-on with anger, while others, like me, opt for the freeze or run away approach, unless I am cornered, when I fight. This works well if your life is under real threat in the moment. An example of this would be walking out in front of a truck or if someone is about to stab you. Your instinct and the response of this part of your brain can save your life.

Despite its good intentions, though, this ancient guardian can lead us astray in the modern world. It feeds on bad news, a trait amplified by today's media landscape. It's constantly on the lookout for potential threats, keeping us in a perpetual state of fight, flight, or freeze, worrying about others' opinions and actions. This can stem from watching news media to office gossiping. The irony lies in the fact that everyone else is grappling with the same concerns: they, too, are worried about what you are thinking about them.

2. Reticular Activating System — The Brain's Bouncer

Imagine the Reticular Activating System as a bouncer at a crowded club, filtering information to prevent overload. It's like standing in a pitch-black warehouse, focused on a path of light leading to the door. This system helps us concentrate on what's crucial while fading out the rest. If you are focusing on getting out of the warehouse via the door, there is a good chance you will miss what's in the darkness. This could be gold and riches but has been faded out.

If our focus is on bad news, the Reticular Activating System diligently serves up more of the same, reinforcing our fears. It adheres to the belief that what we concentrate on is what we want to create, exemplifying the adage, "Where you put your attention, energy flows."

3. Mastering Your Mind's Blueprint

Let's dive into the third crucial component of your mind's intricate machinery — the Results Formula, the true architect of your reality.

This dynamic process follows a clear path: Thoughts spark Feelings, leading to Actions, ultimately producing Results. Many people toss this formula aside, blaming external circumstances for their outcomes.

Now, I want you to take a closer look at this formula. It goes like this: Thoughts → cause → Feeling → cause → Actions → cause → Results. As you reflect on your life and the stories you tell yourself, notice how often you use the word "BECAUSE" to justify why you haven't achieved something or why a desired result hasn't materialized.

For instance, "I didn't get that promotion at work because my boss doesn't like me!"

But here's the twist: instead of pointing fingers at external factors, it's crucial to recognize that our thoughts, triggered by specific moments or events, create feelings that influence our actions and shape the results we experience. It's a continuous cycle governed by the law of cause and effect — our thoughts manifest into reality.

Now, consider this: the problem isn't the boss not liking you; it's the thought itself. Shift that thought to "My boss values my work," and then feel that appreciation. Watch how your actions change with a different energy. Conduct your experiment and see what results you get. Approach it with the energy of already having that promotion, and according to the law described above, you'll get it!

However, challenges arise when negative emotions become ingrained, forming subconscious patterns that dictate our default way of being. Breaking these patterns becomes a conscious struggle between our desires and our body's craving for the familiar emotional fix. This emotional fix sought by the body then triggers the old thought! This is why habits are hard to break, whether it's smoking, alcohol or drug use, or a reliance on adult content. When you try to break free, your subconscious mind, influenced by your body's withdrawals, generates thoughts. Your normal is to have that drink, which momentarily makes you feel better. Then the thoughts of guilt or shame kick in, and we numb them with more of the same addictive behaviour.

Yet, there's hope in this understanding. By grasping how our mind works, we can shed light on the paths to transformation.

In conclusion, the Reptilian Brain, Reticular Activating System, and Results Formula collectively shape our experiences. Unlocking change begins with understanding this blueprint. Armed with this awareness, you wield the power to shift your focus, transform your thoughts, and ultimately reshape the results you create in your life. The journey to your Inner Warrior starts with a profound shift in perspective.

CHAPTER 4

Vision

"Our thoughts shape reality."

To absorb the essence of this chapter, I drew on the wealth of knowledge gained as a Life Mastery Consultant with Mary Morrissey and the Brave Thinking Institute.

Now that we've explored the inner workings of our minds, it's time to wield that knowledge. You've uncovered the truth: our thoughts shape reality. But the crucial question remains
— what thoughts will you choose to nurture and cultivate?

Consider everything around you, from books and pens to tables and chairs. Everything began with an idea — think about your smartphone — the need to communicate across distances, evolving from smoke signals to drums, Morse code, phone lines, cordless phones, cell phones, and finally, the smart device. Each step in communication history began as a thought.

Every thought was an idea that someone took action on and
created in a physical form.

Now that we grasp the law of the cause-and-effect dynamic of our thoughts, let's shift our focus to redesigning our lives. The key lies in crafting the life we desire through the power of imagination. It's about creating rather than merely existing. Reflect on your past focus. Like many, you might have fixated on fears and anxiety after challenges, inadvertently manifesting those very circumstances. The result? A subconscious reality of frustration, anxiety, and fear. During my anxiety-filled drives post-accident, the constant worry of *what if something goes wrong?* became a self-fulfilling prophecy, triggering panic attacks and blackouts.

Remember, nothing changes unless our thinking changes. I had to change the focus of my thinking.

Building on the previous chapter about energy following focus, let's picture the life we truly desire. Most of us meticulously plan holidays or new houses but, surprisingly, few design a vision for their entire life. What would you love in your life?

In the realm of human experience, everything has its opposite

hot and cold, pain and pleasure, dark and light. Likewise, the opposites of fear, anxiety, and scarcity are joy, abundance, gratitude, and love. Your vision should resonate with these higher vibrations.

Ask yourself: What would you love for your life? If

everything in your life magically worked out, what would it look like? Imagine being in love with your life — your health, career, earnings, relationships, and location.

Be aware of the shift in perspective, from these common questions we often ask ourselves for examples.

- What does my family think I can do?
- What does my education say I can do?
- What does my bank account say I can do?
- What do I think I can do?

Instead of the questions above, focus on what you would love to be, do, and have. It's about aligning you with your heart, which will align your life with your power — the Inner Warrior.

One way of achieving this is to craft a powerful vision by falling in love with it. Consider the feelings you'd experience if your dream life were a reality. Imagine the emotions tied to your dream life. Use words like gratitude, happiness, joy, love, flow, ease and grace and add your own words to articulate your beautiful life, using the present tense as you write or speak it.

Gratitude is a potent energy, akin to having your dream on high interest. Incorporate it daily into your vision by starting with the words, "I am happy and grateful now that..." This kick starts your vision in the right vibration, as if it has already happened. However, do leave room for the unexpected — the Inner Warrior might have an even greater gift. Leave your vision open-ended by completing it with this or something even greater still!

In 1995, I stood at a crossroads: did I succumb to my fears by hiding under the covers of that hospital bed and letting life happen to me, or would I pursue my vision of returning to farming? Despite the skepticism around me, including my own doubts and physical limitations, a quiet voice within — my Inner Warrior — asked, "What would you love? Go do that!"

Unbeknownst to me at the time, this vision became my guiding light. It pushed me out of my bed and pulled me to the gym. It gave me the courage to step towards my fears and propelled me to overcome my physical limitations. It took four years, the support of loved ones, and unwavering determination, but I eventually ran and managed my family's 1,100-acre farm.

Pick something you love, anything, and embark on an incredible journey. Even in the seemingly impossible, your vision can be a driving force. At the moment in my hospital bed when I chose going back to the farm, the dream did seem impossible.

Achieving my farming vision was just the beginning. I craved new challenges, actively designing my life rather than letting it unfold. This search led me to incredible experiences like traveling to England, where I learnt to water ski and sail a boat. There was white water rafting in New Zealand, snow skiing, and scuba diving with the sharks in the Napier aquarium - all from a wheelchair. Ultimately, I arrived at the teachings of Mary Morrissey in 2017. Becoming a certified

To explore further, visit my website: http HYPERLINK "http://www.wayneforrest.com/"s://www.wayneforrest.com/

For insights into Mary Morrissey's work and the Brave Thinking Institute, follow this link: http HYPERLINK "http://www.bravethinkinginstitute.com/"s://www.bravethinkinginstitute.com/

consultant under her guidance, I discovered a systematic approach to creating transformative change. Many of the tools and laws I share here, including vision, can be credited to Mary's teachings

CHAPTER 5

Embracing Your Dual Nature Unlocking the Power Within You

"Beyond the realm of the human experience lies an untapped reservoir of power – the Inner Warrior. This innate force, often recognized as intuition, gut sense, or a still, small voice, serves as a beacon of wisdom.

In the intricate tapestry of our existence, we navigate two fundamental aspects of our nature — the human experience and the Inner Warrior within. Let's delve into these realms, understand their dynamics, and harness the extraordinary potential they offer.

The Human Experience: A Journey with Senses

From our first breath to the present day, our lives unfold along a timeline woven with experiences. Birth and, eventually, death mark the boundaries of our human journey. This journey, shaped by our senses,—sight, sound, touch, smell, and taste— immerses us in the rich tapestry of existence. We start as helpless infants, relying entirely on our families for food, warmth, and care, and evolve into survival experts governed by our innate survival brain.

As infants, we communicate not through words but by observing the body language of the enigmatic creatures we called adults. Adapting swiftly, we mirror their interactions, forming connections crucial for our safety and wellbeing. Yet, as we progress through upbringing and the educational system, a shift occurs.

A NASA study from the 1960s highlights a sobering reality: the boundless creativity threshold of 98% for five-year-olds diminishes drastically by adulthood. By 10 years old, it's only at 30%, and it drops another 12% by the age of 15. Adults retain a mere 2% of a creative genius mindset.

The culprit? Conformity. The laughter accompanying any deviation from the norm during our formative years instilled a fear of embarrassment. This fear, etched into our subconscious shaped patterns of behaviour aimed at avoiding a repeat
performance as the class fool.

Whether seeking refuge at the back of the room, adopting the role of the class clown, or withdrawing into ourselves, our actions stem from a primal instinct to evade humiliation. This instinct, often misconstrued as rebellion or naughtiness, conceals a deeper truth: we are attempting to shield ourselves from the sting of past embarrassment. We create an erroneous sense of shame and silently tell ourselves that we aren't good enough.

I worked at a local high school as a mentor for boys aged 13 to
18. The most common method the boys would instigate to get out of class was this so-called 'bad' behaviour in a classroom. The reality is that this is a mechanism of the subconscious brain

avoiding the pain of not-so-good experiences in a classroom from their past. Often, this was because they didn't fit into the academic schooling system.

Our diverse, unique, and individual journeys through life, marked by both positive and negative experiences, contribute to the formation of beliefs. These beliefs, perceived as immutable truths, are the coloured lenses through which we view the world. Yet, it's vital to recognize that these truths, based on past experiences, hold the potential for transformation.

The Inner Warrior: Unleashing Your

Superpower

Beyond the realm of the human experience lies an untapped with your Inner Warrior. Embrace this awakening, for in transforming ourselves, we catalyze change on a global scale.

Dare to envision the change residing within your heart. By reshaping ourselves, we become architects of a better world.

Remember, the power lies within you.

CHAPTER 6

Path to Purpose!

"Your past doesn't define you; it's about who you choose to become from this moment forward. You are the Inner Warrior, embodying unconditional love for yourself and others."

Discovering your purpose can be a transformative journey, and I'm here to guide you through the process. Let's dive into the section and make some improvements for clarity, concision, and style.

If you haven't found your purpose yet, don't worry — I believe this process will lead you there. Let's kick things off with a question that has sparked self-reflection for both my clients and me. It's a bit of hypothetical re-engineering. If, for instance, you were to leave this world tomorrow (which, of course, you won't — picture a long and prosperous life), would you be content with what you've created so far?

Think about it. What's on your bucket list? It could be improved health, a fulfilling relationship, or perhaps more love in the connections you already have. Maybe it's a change in career or a voyage to a distant land. Choose something close to your heart, and let it be the starting point for your journey towards whatever you're meant to create in this life.

Remember, your past doesn't define you; it's about who you choose to become from this moment forward. You are the Inner Warrior, embodying unconditional love for yourself and others.

In my own journey, I've learned that the vision you choose should push you to become a better version of yourself. It should align with the Inner Warrior within you. This process thrives when your dream encourages personal growth, pushing you beyond your comfort zone. It won't work if your goal is too familiar, too easily attainable. We want you to stretch and grow to become a better version of you.

How do you know if you're on the right track? If, during your pursuit, you hear voices in your head telling you that you can't or shouldn't do something, rest assured that you're probably in the right place. A compelling vision should evoke both passion and excitement, as well as fear and excuses as to why you can't. In that contrast lies the perfect vision for you.

Know this: Each of us has something to offer to humanity, or the world we live in. It will be for the betterment of everybody in this collective experience called life.

Courage is taking a step in the direction of your fear of the unknown. If you can, embrace curiosity, trust your Inner Warrior, and let it guide you. It's not your human experience's job to figure out how; that's your Inner Warrior's responsibility. Ask questions, test it out, and watch the magic unfold.

Here are a couple of powerful questions to ask yourself: What can I do from where I am, with what I have, in the direction of my vision? Show me my next step. What would it take to become the person in my vision? Trust your Inner Warrior, and let it show you the way to your dream.

Imagine if you knew that the intelligence breathing life into you has your back. As Albert Einstein said, "The most important decision we make is whether we believe we live in a friendly or hostile universe." Surrendering and letting go of the need to know the how can make life easier.

So, are you pushing, or are you flowing? Life is meant to be cool and easy, like a river, and it flows when we live in alignment with our Inner Warrior. Challenge your human conditioning, which tends to push or fight hard for what we want. Yes, be rigorous, work smart, by taking those Inner Warrior scary action steps, but leave the 'how' to your inner power, the Inner Warrior.

Your only task is to build a better relationship with your Inner Warrior and become the person in your vision. Trust that your Inner Warrior holds all the answers to your questions and solutions to your problems. Be curious, ask lots of questions, and test it out. Some answers may come from your human experience but within them lies your inner power, waiting to both scare and excite you.

This process involves creating a clear vision of what you would love and ensuring it pushes you out of your comfort zone. Learn to listen to your Inner Warrior, as courage is needed to step into the unknown. Your path won't unfold exactly as you imagine it; your Inner Warrior loves to surprise you with its unique expression of your vision, which is always better and more surprising than you could ever imagine, especially given the collective human experience that we get to share.

You'll know when you're in alignment with your Inner Warrior. Life becomes easier, and synchronicities unfold unexpectedly. Things and people fall into place, helping you create a life filled with your envisioned purpose.

CHAPTER 7

Decide for Your Life!

"Make committed decisions for your vision, even in tough times. If you can picture it in your mind and truly love it, then it's possible."

Nothing changes if we don't change, and if you want change, you have to commit to changing what you do. The decisions we make today will ultimately shape who we become tomorrow.

There's something magical about deciding for the vision you've created. Energy moves and rearranges itself to rush in and fill the vacuum created by the vision. This alignment with your Inner Warrior's dream triggers a series of events. Opportunities and people emerge for the realization of your vision. Synchronicities happen, and everything flows, similar to a stream cascading over a waterfall.

Yet, amid the flow, we often panic!

"Whoa! Slow down, let's swim away from the waterfall!" In essence, we halt the flow and swim away from the vision. It sounds crazy, right? But we've all done it.

What lies beyond the waterfall? It's either your vision or a crucial step towards it. Yet, sometimes fear creeps in, causing us to panic and divert from the stream. We forget that surrendering and trusting the current is essential for progress.

Trusting your Inner Warrior means relinquishing control, which doesn't feel natural to us. Our human experience has taught us to be cautious, to watch out for danger. As we can't see what's on the other side, fear of the unknown takes hold.

Many of us encounter multiple waterfalls on the stream to our vision. We might commit at the first and second waterfalls, but when faced with the biggest and scariest ones, we may panic and jump out of the stream altogether. We dip our toes into a new stream, starting a new vision.

This is why repeatedly committing to the vision is crucial. Examples from my life include paying a deposit for a course without having all the money or selling our house to move across the country without a confirmed place to live.

Living in a wheelchair adds another layer of challenge: not knowing where we'll live is tougher. But these are just facts, challenges, and conditions in my life. They don't define who I am or what I can do; only my belief can.

Consider my story during my accident. I had a choice: wallow in self-pity or make a life for myself. I listened to my Inner Warrior whispering, "What would you love?" Choosing to go back to my farm was a commitment that rearranged things in my favour. People, opportunities, and things aligned to make my dream a reality.

One significant support was my personal carer, Jen Stoddart, who lived only minutes away from my farm. Married to a local farmer herself, she was a physio with experience in spinal injuries. Think how rare that is, in the middle of nowhere.

Jen helped me daily, and her knowledge, coaching, accountability, support and expertise were crucial in regaining movement and strength. Eleven months to regain movement in one of my arms! This is the power of making a decision for your vision. I honestly believe that without Jen in my corner at that time I would not have achieved the strength or the ability to transfer from my wheelchair to a vehicle, or drive, plus the many other personal goals that gave me different levels of independence.

Committing to my vision made running my farm possible.

So, make committed decisions for your vision, even in tough times. If you can picture it in your mind and truly love it, then it's possible. As Goethe wrote, "At the moment of commitment, the entire Universe conspires to assist you". By committing to what it is in your heart, your Inner Warrior will conspire to assist you!

CHAPTER 8

Breaking Free from Limiting Beliefs

"Your Inner Warrior knows no limits; it's your human nature that casts doubts."

Your Inner Warrior knows no limits; it's your human nature that casts doubts. In this chapter we'll explore the dance between the human experience and the Inner Warrior, the yin and yang within all of us.

Embrace curiosity as you journey through this chapter. Picture your life as a game where you are the hero. Every compelling story also needs a villain or some kind of betrayal, or there wouldn't be the need for a hero. In this game of life, you are the hero, and your limited thoughts play the role of villains.

Everyone grapples with limiting thoughts on this quantum plane called life. These beliefs hold the key to unlocking more love in our lives. Celebrate your limited thoughts, for they reveal where we need more love, allowing us to rise up and become the hero of our own story.

Love, often misunderstood, takes various forms, from the love of sports to the love of chocolate, and the complexity of intimate relationships. What if everything is love? Yes, even the challenging parts of our lives. What if everything is an expression of love or a call for love?

Drawing inspiration from the Course of Miracles, rooted in ancient texts from the Dead Sea Scrolls, we must distinguish between expressing love, (what I am calling unconditional love) and seeking it. We often unskillfully seek love to try to make ourselves feel better.

The limiting beliefs are a side-effect of the deeper-rooted

trauma that has created doubt in your true self.

We often then look for love outside ourselves to fix the problem. It only gives a temporary fix until, again, someone or something triggers the pain. We then reinforce that belief of the limiting story we tell ourselves. These beliefs will limit the results you create. To break this circle, first become aware of the pattern, which is trigger — belief — reaction.

Consider Kody's journey, a client. Kody is a well-built man with a tough exterior masking unresolved anger. Through self-reflection, he traced the roots of his anger to childhood, discovering a protective mechanism. Of getting angry to protect himself, his words were, "If I hurt others before I get hurt myself, I can protect myself".

We did an exercise where I got him to look at that anger, where it was in his body and what colour it was. It was in the pit of his stomach and the colour red. I then asked him to connect with his

Inner Warrior and visualize unconditional love for something in his life, which was his children. I then asked him where this was in his body. It was in his heart. He transformed his anger by growing the colour of his love throughout his body and overtaking the colour of his anger.

Kody's Inner Warrior has a great sense of humour, with the colour of pinkish-white love. Everybody's colour is different, as mine is golden-white with flecks of purple, and I can't help but wonder if the harder your outer shell the softer the colour. One thing is for sure: for him to own it, it has to be sacred and aligned to his power, the Inner Warrior. He looked at his pain that he was turning into anger, acknowledged it, and now he is breaking free from the limiting belief. This is a practice of growing your awareness, one moment at a time, if it isn't already there. It will come. Trust the process outlined in this book.

Acknowledge your own limiting thoughts and stories. Practice self-love and awareness, even in discomfort. As you step into your higher self, embracing the vision that stretches your growth, confront the villain — your limiting story.
It's important to note that if you stretch into becoming a better version of yourself, your villain will emerge. The choice is then yours. Will you be the victim or the hero? If you choose victimhood,

you will simply repeat the game until you become the hero.

Remember, there are two types of love: the expression of love (your Inner Warrior) and the call for love, manifesting as anger, anxiety, sadness, depression and any other limiting feelings. Be aware of the limiting thoughts and stories, acknowledge them, and remind yourself of the truth — you are the hero in your game, and you are choosing unconditional love.

In this moment, wrap your younger self in your version of love, whether it's pinkish-white, golden-white with flecks of purple, or any colour that resonates with you. Release the human experiences that weren't yours to carry, understanding that others may have unknowingly passed them down. This doesn't mean you excuse their bad behaviour and if it's hurting you or someone else, get out of there and get help. You can give unconditional love and send them on their way, but always prioritize your own safety.

By understanding, acknowledging, and choosing love, you break free from the cycle of limiting beliefs, leveling up into another level of your life's game.

CHAPTER 9

Understanding Human Experience and the Inner Warrior

"What's the secret to living a life filled with joy, happiness, and love? It begins with recognizing that you are the Inner Warrior, the spirit within the human having this profound experience."

Let's dive into the distinction between the two concepts of the human experience and the Inner Warrior with the aim to simplify this for you all.

I refer to the higher nature as the Inner Warrior to make it relatable and straightforward. This term, I believe, will resonate with many of you, and some of you will prefer other names like Spirit, higher Self, Universe and God. Depending on your belief system, you can call it whatever you want. What we can agree on is that there is some kind of intelligence breathing in us all.

Within our powerful spiritual side, we possess the various natures of the Inner Warrior. I aim to present these concepts in a way that's accessible to beginners and those already journeying towards awareness of consciousness, known as love.

So, what's the secret to living a life filled with joy, happiness, and love? It begins with recognizing that you are the Inner Warrior, the spirit within the human having this profound experience. This is why people say we are spiritual beings having a human experience and not the other way around.

Albert Einstein says it this way: "Energy cannot be created or destroyed; it can only be changed from one form to another. Everything is energy and that is all there is to it. Match the frequency of the reality you want and you cannot help but get that reality. It can be no other way."

This energy is the Inner Warrior and I believe you don't need to take my word on it. Stay curious, exploring, and questioning everything while believing in nothing, and you'll inevitably arrive at this truth. It's crucial to understand that neither side of our nature — Human experience nor the Inner Warrior — is inherently good or bad. Both are necessary to create, build, and experience life to its fullest potential in the physical realm.

However, imbalance is often an issue. Many of us find ourselves immersed in too much Human experience and not enough Inner Warrior presence in our lives. As awareness grows, we begin to tap into our Inner Warrior, fostering a balance that spreads like a ripple throughout humanity, fostering more unconditional love.

Let's simplify further. Consider the Inner Warrior as synonymous with unconditional love, a perspective that sees abundance in everything, recognizing your perfection and completeness. It's a love that gives without expecting anything in return, characterized by generosity and compassion.

Yet, grasping this concept can be challenging, especially when faced with immediate survival needs like food and shelter. In such circumstances, it is hard to see your opportunities or even the possibility of something better. Our brains operate on a loop of scarcity, reinforcing the law of cause and effect by focusing on the real need in that moment. (Which could be as simple as food and shelter.) This cycle, described in Matthew 25:29, seems harsh, but it reflects our natural inclination.

"For to everyone who has will more be given, and he will have abundance; but from him who has not, even what he has will be taken away".

This seems tough because the old brain focus is on what can harm us, which naturally works against us by creating more of the same.

In reality, the world doesn't suffer from a lack of resources (not yet, anyway) but rather from a deficit of unconditional love, either from greed or the lack of circulation. The root of issues like greed, scarcity, and competition lie in our conditioned responses, the result of our human experience or ego. We can label this aspect of ourselves as conditional love, highlighting the conditioned nature of human behaviour.

Increasing awareness of our actions and

motivations, whether they stem from conditional or unconditional love, can lead to profound shifts. Many of these patterns were ingrained in us during childhood as we sought security and affection. For instance, consider how we often resort to conditional love tactics to get what we desire, be it from our children, partners, or colleagues.

The Inner Warrior, on the other hand, uplifts others and oneself, recognizing and fostering inherent power. Healthy competition arises when we use someone else's success as inspiration to improve our own lives. This mindset mirrors the approach of figures like Jesus, not in a religious context, but more simply because he was someone who epitomized living in unconditional love as the Inner Warrior.

Consider the story of Jesus and the paralytic. The story goes like this. The first person to enter the pool when the waters were stirred up would supposedly be cured of his or her ailment. But the paralytic tells Jesus he can never get into the water quickly enough. Despite the man's physical limitations, Jesus saith unto him, Rise, take up thy bed, and walk. And immediately the man was made whole, and took up his bed, and walked" (verses 5–9). Let's unpack this for a moment. Jesus saw beyond him, encouraging him to embrace his potential. Similarly, He persuaded the man to believe in his potential, the power (the Inner Warrior), where everything is possible.

This story was told to me by my mentor, Mary Morrissey, and it made me confront my own limiting beliefs following the accident. The doctor at the time told me I would never walk again. I took that as truth and thus capped my potential. Don't get me wrong. I was determined to defy expectations and achieve remarkable feats, but I was always limited within that belief.

I have created an amazing life. I have a beautiful wife, who's my best friend, four kids and five grandchildren, thus far. I have run a farm, traveled the world, and moved across the country, all in the pursuit of my dreams.

I share these experiences not to boast but to illustrate that even in moments of triumph, limiting beliefs can persist. Yet, by embracing unconditional love, we unlock limitless possibilities. Yes, doubts and fears may arise — the words come to mind of what if I fail? — but by grounding ourselves in unconditional love in that moment, we align with our true essence, paving the way for a happier, effortless life.

Let's embrace the journey of self-discovery rooted in unconditional love, where every action and decision comes from our true power and essence. As we do so, we'll find joy, abundance, and fulfillment beyond measure.

CHAPTER 10

Release the Old for the New!

"Unconditional love is where true strength and resilience lies. You only have to witness a man being authentic with vulnerability to feel the power in that."

Imagine yourself as a ball of energy, contained within a vessel already brimming with experiences and emotions. If we seek to infuse this energy with more unconditional love, we must first make room by releasing some of the old, conditional love.

Let's start by shedding the layers of anger, frustration, and limiting beliefs that we all carry. Before we delve into this, though, let's address the elephant in the room. This talk of love, whether unconditional or conditional, might seem a world away from the mindset of our younger version selves, especially in a time when displaying anything other than macho bravado was seen as weakness. I understand this might be uncomfortable for many guys out there, but if you can push past that discomfort and embrace this concept, you'll discover a profound power within it. Unconditional love is where true strength and resilience lies. You only have to witness a man being authentic with vulnerability to feel the power in that. I've found that the more open and vulnerable I am about these ideas, the more I attract other men who are eager to engage in these discussions. It fosters a genuine, deep connection that feels incredibly real.

However, the true transformative power lies in replacing conditional love, which often manifests as anger, frustration or sadness, with unconditional love within ourselves. Our energy vessel is constantly full, but some of that energy weighs us down. In fact, the word 'disease' is simply dis-ease in your body. Replacing this heavy, conditional love energy with the freeing and lightness of unconditional love can have significant health benefits. This often entails forgiveness, whether forgiving ourselves or others for past actions or inactions. We all have someone who, when they cross our minds, ignites a storm of resentment and hurt. But this isn't about them; it's about cultivating more unconditional love within ourselves to lead happier, more fulfilling lives.

We must find a way to separate the emotion from the act, whether it's something we did or something that was done to us that creates the energy and frequency of feelings like hurt, betrayal, guilt, shame, or anger. These emotional energies create acid in the body, eating away at you and fostering dis- ease. It's been likened to drinking poison and hoping the person who hurt you dies. I have found personally changing the perception of why or how something happened can be a powerful tool in this process. It can take some practise, though, to acquire a belief that everything is for us and not just happening to us. There are different forgiveness practices out there, so do a little research and find one that helps you release the emotion and replace it in your energy ball with unconditional love for yourself.

Even I still find myself triggered from time to time, perhaps by my wife inadvertently pressing on past pains, but the more I practice forgiveness, the quicker I can let go of that heavy energy. I can feel it weighing on my chest or knotting my stomach, but with my newfound awareness, it no longer feels like the norm. Through self-awareness and embracing unconditional love, I've learned to quiet those triggers and foster deeper understanding and harmony.

It's essential to realize that forgiveness isn't a one-time thing; it should be a daily practice, much like brushing your teeth. And it's not about absolving guilt, obligation, or punishment from the other person or situation, but rather acknowledging past hurts and traumas and releasing their hold on us. I recently had a conversation with a client who offered a beautiful perspective on forgiveness. He doesn't see it as pardoning the wrongdoer; instead, it's about acknowledging the past pain, thanking it for its lessons, and enveloping those past versions of ourselves in love and light.

He likened it to comforting a crying child, but within us, reassuring them that they're not alone and guiding them towards healing. With this understanding, we can extend that same compassion to ourselves, recognizing that we are our own Inner Warriors.

For my client, forgiveness was about transcending the hurt and embracing the unconditional love within himself. It's about recognizing that the wounded child within us often dictates our reactions to triggers. Once we grasp this, we can choose to respond from the perspective of the Inner Warrior, showering that wounded child within us with unconditional love and assurance.

This is the process of releasing conditional love from our energy ball and replacing it with the boundless love of the Inner Warrior. And the best part. You can start right now. That's the magic of unconditional love — it's always within reach.

CHAPTER 11

Unraveling the Tangled Web of Self-Conditioned Love

"It all began with a narrative whispered in the corridors of my mind, a relentless echo of never being quite good enough."

Let me share my story with you, a tale woven through the lens of hindsight, 29 years post-accident, from where I stand today, the threads of my past intricately connected, revealing a story deeply rooted in a perpetual sense of inadequacy.

It all began with a narrative whispered in the corridors of my mind, a relentless echo of never being quite good enough. For me, this manifested as an insatiable drive to outshine everyone else, particularly in areas where I excelled.

One such arena was rugby, a passion for which I can't pinpoint the origin, though I suspect it gestated during my school years. Academic struggles cast me as the classroom misfit, branded as 'dumb' by teachers and peers alike. Such labels erode confidence and breed social isolation; I became a solitary figure, wary of trusting others for fear of betrayal and judgment.

Everything changed at 17 when I switched schools. No longer the butt of every joke, I seized rugby as my conduit to acceptance. Lunch breaks were dominated by Scragg, a brutal form of rugby that left torn shirts and bruised egos in its wake. But amidst the chaos, I found friendship and respect, I had a large group of friends who were boys and girls, a stark departure from my previous social alienation of an all-boys boarding school.

Yet beneath the façade of strength lay a crippling self-doubt, reinforced by a callous remark from a math teacher at the new school, a reminder that my intellect was suspect. But I buried my insecurities deep, masking them with bravado and athleticism.

Fast forward eight years, and I appeared the epitome of stability: married, father of twins, and carving out a living as a farmer and sheep shearer. But beneath the veneer of adulthood lay a foundation built on shaky ground.

The day of my accident began like any other, with a friend visiting from abroad. Eager to impress, I took to the rugby field, driven by a subconscious need for validation. Assigned captaincy in the absence of key players, I played with reckless abandon, heedless of the risks although, to be truthful, this wasn't unusual.

Then, in a split-second decision, I threw myself into the fray, determined to maintain possession at any cost. But fate had other plans; the collision that ensued left me with a dislocated vertebra and a shattered illusion of invincibility.

Reflecting now, I see the tragic irony of my story:

a quest for validation through physical prowess that ultimately led to my undoing. My refusal to yield stemmed not from courage, but from a desperate need to prove my worth.

But this isn't just my story — it's a narrative to which many can relate. We all seek validation in different ways, be it through sports, academics, or social acceptance. But beneath the surface lies a common thread of insecurity, a belief that we're not enough as we are.

For me, the journey to self-acceptance began with a harsh awakening, but it needn't be so for others. By acknowledging our insecurities and relinquishing the need for external validation, we open ourselves to a world of abundance and joy.

My accident was a catalyst for change. It's helping me heal the pain in my heart from not feeling like I was enough, as crazy as that might sound. It was the vehicle to my own healing!

But it needn't take such drastic measures to prompt self- reflection. Each of us has the power to rewrite our stories, to embrace our flaws and celebrate our uniqueness.

So, I ask you: are you ready to listen? Are you ready to rewrite your story, free from the constraints of self-doubt? The choice is yours.

CHAPTER 12

Manifestation Demystified

"Our thoughts are the architects of our existence."

"Let gratitude, belief, and action be your guiding stars."

Manifestation, the art of shaping your reality through thought and emotion, is a profound force in our lives, whether we acknowledge it or not. As my mentor, Mary Morrissey, often emphasizes, our thoughts are the architects of our existence. I firmly believe that, as humans, we are not just observers but active participants in the creation of our own lives.

Consider this scenario. When you choose to spend the day in bed, hiding under the covers, you're essentially manifesting a day of rest. That's because where we focus our attention, our energy follows. The thoughts we dwell on, especially when infused with emotion, tend to materialize into our reality over time.

Take illness, for example. Sure, you might catch a bug that's going around, but whether it actually makes you sick can often be traced back to your mindset. Negative thoughts weaken your immune system, making you more susceptible to illness. If you constantly tell yourself you're always getting sick, guess what? You're likely to get sick more often. Conversely, believing in your robust health can serve as a protective shield against illness.

Let me share a personal example. Despite having a permanent suprapubic catheter due to my past injury, I rarely suffer from urinary tract infections

(UTIs). Why? Because I firmly believe I am immune to them. Even when I spend time with a sick family member, I quickly dismiss any notion of falling ill myself. I refuse to entertain thoughts of weakness or vulnerability, knowing that my body and environment are inherently resilient. If I entertain a thought of weakness for too long, and I have on occasion, I have a great chance of getting sick. During the 2020 pandemic, I had so many people worried about my health that I entertained the thought with the emotion of fear and I did fall ill, even though mildly.

Mastering manifestation doesn't require perfection. It's about gradually shifting your mindset from replacing negative emotion to positive, from doubt to belief. Have you ever noticed those individuals who boast about never getting sick? They're not just lucky. They've tapped into the power of their own thoughts to shape their reality.

So, how do you harness this power for yourself? It starts with identifying what you truly desire by asking yourself, what would I love? Then you craft a vivid vision with clarity and detail for your life. This vision should evoke a deep sense of longing within you, igniting a burning desire to see it come to fruition.

Next comes grateful expectation, a state of mind

where you don't hope or want for your vision to manifest but fully expect it to become a reality. It's about embracing a mindset of gratitude as if your desired outcome has already materialized. This aligns your energy with the frequency of love and abundance, which is the frequency of creation itself, making manifestation feel effortless.

But manifestation isn't wishful thinking. It's knowing that it has been ordered and is on its way and when we know something is happening, then it must require action from us. Surround yourself with people who embody the reality you seek to create. By immersing yourself in their energy and adopting their mindset, you'll naturally begin to align with the vibration of your desired outcome. This is why they say if you want to be a millionaire you should surround yourself with millionaire friends.

Remember, obstacles may arise along the way, but trust in your vision and stay committed to your path. Just like a river flowing towards the ocean, let the current of your desires carry you forward, knowing that every challenge is simply a detour to learning something on the journey to your dreams.

So, as you navigate the waters of manifestation, let gratitude, belief, and action be your guiding stars. With these tools at your disposal, you have the power to design a life that not only meets your expectations but exceeds them. Embrace the journey, for the destination is already within your grasp.

CHAPTER 13

The Process!

*"Success isn't just a stroke of luck.
It's a methodical journey upon which
anyone can embark."*

Success isn't just a stroke of luck. It's a methodical journey upon which anyone can embark. This process has been utilized by leaders, athletes, entrepreneurs, and everyday people like you and me, in some cases without even realizing it. Take myself, for instance. When I made the decision to return to farming after my accident, I didn't realize I was following a structured path to success. It wasn't until years later when I came across Mary Morrissey and her teachings on DreamBuilding that I understood the system I had been using. If I can do it, so can you.

We all possess the same infinite, boundless potential, regardless of our academic achievements or qualifications. But by all means if your vision requires you to get accreditations, go do it. Each of us has unique strengths and skills that we should harness to our advantage, recognizing that this process isn't just applicable to our individual lives but to humanity as a whole. That fills me with hope for the future. Every challenge we encounter as humans inherently carries a solution; we simply need to ask the right questions and approach them from a different perspective.

As Albert Einstein famously said, "You cannot solve a problem with the same mind that created it." This quote resonates deeply with me, signifying the importance of shifting our mindset towards envisioning the desired outcome rather than dwelling on the problem itself. By embodying the vibration of the person in our vision we aspire to become and focusing on gratitude and unconditional love, we set ourselves on a path of transformation.

However, not everyone may be ready to embrace this journey alongside us. And that's okay. Everyone is on their own unique path, and while some may not be prepared to elevate their vibration to match yours, by working on yourself you will create a ripple effect and, although you might never know it, others may find inspiration in your journey.

Now, let's delve into the five steps of this transformative process:

1. **Vision:** Clearly articulate your vision in the present tense, embodying the reality of it happening now. Ask yourself, "What would I love?"

2. **Visualization:** Immerse yourself in the feeling of achieving your vision. Visualize it upon waking, during the day, and before sleep. Keep the flame of desire burning bright with gratitude and anticipation.

3.   Acknowledging the Inner Child: Recognize the voice of the triggered child within who is fearful of stepping out of the comfort zone. Celebrate its presence and shower it with unconditional love while acknowledging its origin in past trauma.

4.   Embracing the Inner Warrior: Identify with your Inner Warrior, the embodiment of abundance, courage, and innate potential. Take inspired action towards your vision, repeating and reinforcing this mindset.

5.   Courageous Action: Step boldly into your vision, inhabiting the spirit of the Inner Warrior. Trust in the process and expect the desired outcome with unwavering faith.

I'd like to leave you with a quote that has deeply resonated with me: "Don't ask what the world needs. Ask what makes you come alive and go do it. Because what the world needs is people who have come alive." — Howard Thurman.

This quote encapsulates the essence of living a fulfilling life

— following our passions and embracing what brings us joy. Take my wife, for example, who found immense happiness in being with her horses but felt societal pressure to pursue a more traditional career. It took a shift in perspective for her to realize that by immersing herself in what she loves, she not only finds fulfillment but also attracts abundance into her life.

Ultimately, life is about creating, growing, and expanding. Don't wait for opportunities to come knocking; seize them with the fervour of your Inner Warrior. Embrace your true nature, fall in love with every aspect of your existence, and watch as the universe aligns to support your journey. Here's to love, growth, and the limitless potential within each of us

Manufactured by Amazon.ca
Acheson, AB

14387656R00046